1

A Complete Look at CFS and Fibromyalgia

The Syndromes of Fatigue and Body Pain

© 2010 By: James M. Lowrance

TABLE OF CONTENTS

A Complete Look at CFS and Fibromyalgia

INTRODUCTION

Chronic Fatigue Syndrome and Fibromyalgia affect millions of Americans and many millions more worldwide. The Debilitating fatigue and joint/muscle pain these syndromes cause can seriously reduce the quality-of-life for those who experience them. Aspects of these illnesses can include the following.

• Viral, fungal and bacterial components
• hormonal and nutritional deficiencies
• adrenal fatigue (low cortisol and/or DHEA levels)

Chronic Fatigue Syndrome and Fibromyalgia are real illnesses recognized by the U.S. National Institutes of Health and other World Health Organizations. While they are separately recognized illnesses, they have 75% crossover similarities. It is my hope that this book will provide an informative general educational resource for readers wishing to learn more about these very real, life-changing illnesses.

A Complete Look at CFS and Fibromyalgia

CHAPTER ONE

The Symptoms of Chronic Fatigue Syndrome and Fibromyalgia

Since many symptoms of CFS and Fibromyalgia are in-common with both syndromes, the symptom list that follows will be an equal possibility for being experienced with both syndromes. With the two major characteristic symptoms that distinguish between the two syndromes being "fatigue" (CFS) and "body pain" (Fibromyalgia). Both can be present in each illness but if one or the other is prominent, this helps to distinguish between them.

• Fatigue (ongoing and following exertion)
• Joint/muscle aches & tender points (with the absence of redness or swelling of joints)
• Neurological symptoms (i.e. headaches, tremors, dizziness and sensory changes)
• Emotional symptoms (i.e. anxiety and/or depression)
• Cognitive problems (i.e. difficulty concentrating and short-term memory loss)

The following two stories are fictitious examples, written by me – the author, to serve as examples of how one might discover that they are suffering from CFS and/or Fibromyalgia.

Fictitious Scenario for Fibromyalgia:

Jane Doe says:
"When I was in my mid thirties, I started having some joint pain that started in my knees and I thought it was from doing too much gardening on my hands and knees. I didn't think much about it until I noticed more muscle stiffness and aches as months and years went by. One morning I woke up and I felt this stiffness throughout my body and began to wonder if I might have some kind of arthritis affecting me.

I started taking pain relief - over the counter medicines which helped some but the muscle pain continued to worsen overall and after a while I was taking the highest dose of brand name pain medicines you could buy off the shelf. I knew then it was time to see a doctor and ask about tests for arthritis.

The doctor I ended up with told me my problem was just from aging and going through the menopause age but I knew it was far more serious and I asked him if tests for arthritis might be a good idea. He told me that without any joint swelling or redness around my joints, these type tests were of no purpose. I went home that day greatly disappointed because my hope was in being prescribed something to help with the pain that had spread all over by body. I was watching a television documentary about a man who went through almost exactly what I was going through and it got my attention when they diagnosed him with fibromyalgia.

I made a new appointment with a different doctor whose specialty was diabetes but who was known for being more thorough with patients. He listened to my story and started a physical exam of me and he started to press his finger in different areas of my muscles and this caused remarkable pain on some of these spots. He didn't even have to ask me when I had pain because I would jump and wince when some of these spots were pressed against.

He had an expression of recognition on his face at that point and when I questioned him he said that it was almost certain I had fibromyalgia because I had at least 11 tender spots around different joints in my body.

I was relieved in one sense and scared in another. He had me get blood tests for arthritis and autoimmune problems and these were negative I had a mild elevation in inflammation shown on the test results and a mildly high creatinine kinase blood level which indicated mild muscle damage with a small degree of inflammation. He told me that many fibromyalgia patients have no positive lab findings but that my physical exam and medical history was certain for my having it. My doctor is treating me with analgesic drugs for pain and inflammation and he has me on a low dose of anti-seizure medication which also helps with pain. I may also have an antidepressant added to my treatment if these other drugs are not completely successful in relieving the pain. At this point I'm just hoping for the best with the treatment I'm already on."

Fictitious Scenario for Chronic Fatigue Syndrome:

John Doe says:
"As a college student in the 1990s, I woke up one morning and literally, that day found I was totally exhausted and drained of energy. This continued for months, in fact after six months the fatigue was still not letting up. I just barely functioned enough to complete my required studies and tests. I felt so drained after cramming for tests or taking them that it took me two days to rest up from them. I went to the campus clinic and was told I had depression but I knew better. My mom set an appointment for me with her doctor and he performed tests on me for 3 months and I mean for everything under the sun that might be wrong with me.

The test findings that stuck out were my virus counts which were through the roof. I had an Epstein-Barr virus number in the 100s and an HV6 virus count also in the 100s. The doctor said this showed that my immune system was not functioning normally and he started me on immune boosting drugs and vitamins.

A Complete Look at CFS and Fibromyalgia

I improved about 40% after a little over four months and have since improved about 60% and hoping for more improvement. Chronic Fatigue Syndrome is real and let no one tell you otherwise. My doctor told me that some people heal from it while others only recover partially and have symptoms for many years. He assured me that younger people who get CFS recover better and more completely than do middle age people and older."

CHAPTER TWO

Conditions That Cause Mild Adrenal Insufficiency

Adrenal insufficiency is a condition in which the adrenal glands do not produce enough hormones to aid in regulating the body's metabolism, stress coping, controlling inflammation and sexual functioning. The main adrenal hormone that becomes low with this condition is "cortisol," and when low levels are detected in a person, it is sometimes referred to as "hypocortisolemia". Full blown adrenal insufficiency is referred to as "Addison's Disease." There are, however, milder forms of adrenal dysfunction as listed below.

Post Traumatic Stress Disorder. This condition, abbreviated PTSD, is a traumatic stress-caused condition that is also considered to be an anxiety disorder. People experience the onset of this disorder as a result of severe traumatizing experiences, such as car accidents, acts of violence that are perpetrated upon them, the sudden loss of a loved one or having been in active combat during wartime.

The severe shock caused to the body from such incidents can cause the glands regulating adrenal hormone output to become "blunted", meaning they begin to function at a sub-normal level. While their adrenal hormones may remain within normal limits, they will be at lowest normal (borderline low), which causes them to have an inability to cope with stressors.

Research studies on PTSD that are published by reputable medical groups (including the U.S. National Institutes of Health) state that low cortisol levels found in patients with this disorder contributes to their symptoms of anxiety, insomnia and flashbacks, meaning they may mentally relive their traumatic experiences repeatedly.

In controlled test studies, using cortisol supplementation to treat PTSD patients, results showed that symptoms were reduced significantly by carefully monitored physiological dosing to increase their level of the low stress hormone.

Chronic Fatigue Syndrome (CFS). This condition has also been found to cause a low level of the stress hormone cortisol evidenced by analyzing the blood and urine cortisol levels in people who experience the illness. Research studies on CFS have repeatedly confirmed this fact and have also found that patients report that they were experiencing chronic or sudden severe stress just before the onset of the illness. This would mean that CFS is very possibly also a stress-related condition that causes the adrenal hormone regulating glands in the body to become blunted.

The U.S. National Institutes of Health released a report in October of 1996, in which they found through a controlled study, that cortisol supplementation/replacement in patients with CFS had a benefit but was found to be short-lived. Afterward, some patients began experiencing a more severe form of adrenal suppression, meaning it caused a worsening of their adrenal insufficiency after a few weeks on the cortisol replacement drug.

13

Fibromyalga Syndrome (FMS). Being very similar to CFS, Fibromyalgia also has chronic fatigue as a major symptom. The aspect that sets this illness apart from CFS is the widespread body pain that is not found to be as prominent in CFS patients. Despite this fact, researchers studying both illnesses have found them to have 75% crossover similarities. This includes the fact that FMS patients often report chronic stress as being a factor in their development of the illness.

A number of research studies have also found cortisol levels to be low in FMS patients and controlled trials of cortisol supplementation have been conducted to determine if there would be a benefit for these patients.

The findings were similar to those found when supplementing CFS patients with cortisol hormone replacement and while some patients improved, the long-term risks for using the drug (i.e. adrenal suppression) did not merit establishing it as a medically recognized treatment for FMS.

A Complete Look at CFS and Fibromyalgia

Adrenal Fatigue. This sub-clinical form of adrenal insufficiency is still not recognized widely by the medical community, although certain types of doctors recognize the disorder, including MDs who practice holistic treatments, Naturopaths and Osteopathic Physicians.

With this condition which is also referred to as "low adrenal reserves" and "adrenal exhaustion", many of the symptoms found in CFS and FMS are not present, including joint and muscle pain and other inflammatory problems in the body.

Adrenal Fatigue is strictly a condition causing mild to moderate fatigue and reduced stress tolerance. Some medical sources are stating that adrenal fatigue that is prolonged and not treated, through proper rest, improved diet, adrenal boosting natural supplements and reducing contributing stressors, may result in the condition becoming a precursor (a pre-condition) to CFS and FMS.

While the conditions I have listed are commonly found to cause mild adrenal insufficiency, other conditions can also be a cause or contributing factor. This includes other chronic and inflammatory diseases that contribute to increased stress levels in the body.

CHAPTER THREE

The Role of Adrenal Fatigue in Illnesses

Many Doctors only recognize the most severe form of adrenal hypo-function called Addison's' Disease or full blown adrenal insufficiency and they base whether or not a patient has this potentially life-threatening form, via the "ACTH Stimulation Test". The problem is that many people have a less severe form called adrenal fatigue or adrenal exhaustion and though these patients nearly always pass the ACTH Stimulation Test, they still have inadequate adrenal hormone levels that show up clearly on lab tests and though it is not life-threatening, it still causes concerning symptoms that can seriously affect quality of life.

The National Institutes of Health, while studying Chronic Fatigue Syndrome, found "low cortisol" to be a factor in it as well and in one of these studies, they made this statement; "Doctors have long known that even subtle deficiencies in cortisol can be associated with lethargy and fatigue."

The "NIAMS" (arthritis etc...) Department of the National Institutes of Health also recognizes low cortisol in Fibromyalgia. Other studies they've published on the PubMed/National Libraries of Medicine website, also recognize low cortisol in PTSD (Post Traumatic Stress Disorders). The fact is that adrenal fatigue can be a factor in these and other chronic diseases/syndromes but other times is stress-related or not related to anything specific.

The most important thing, if you feel you may have adrenal fatigue, is to be tested for it because other hormone imbalances and illnesses cause similar symptoms. Some pharmacies are now carrying saliva hormone testing kits, including ones that test adrenal hormones (cortisol), so you may want to check for the availability of these in your area. If they are not available locally, one can order them online using the search term "adrenal hormone saliva test kits".

The passion I have in the area of adrenal fatigue, besides experiencing it myself, as part of CFS and thyroid disease is the fact that far too many studies and reputable organizations recognize it.

A Complete Look at CFS and Fibromyalgia

This includes the "Fibro & Fatigue Centers", located in 15 states that are staffed by Board Certified MDs from just about every field of medicine. This plus the fact that there are U.S. Government health studies that have also concluded that there are low-cortisol syndromes or well established sub-clinical forms of adrenal hypo-function, that could all be referred to under the term; "adrenal fatigue".

CHAPTER FOUR

Cortisol & DHEA Supplements for Adrenal Fatigue

Over the past four years, I have written a lot on the subject of mild hypo-cortisolism that is found in different conditions, that for lack of another well-established term, we call "adrenal fatigue" but it is often during the research I'm doing at any given time for articles etc..., that I find often, that many in the medical community, still do not recognize mild forms of adrenal insufficiency and they do not believe that adrenal fatigue syndromes exist.

I actually hope Doctors or knowledgeable people of any type will make a suggestion for a name that doesn't come across as bogus and at the same time, if they don't believe sub-clinical forms of adrenal hypo-cortisolism exist, to also explain why all of the research articles that describe it, are somehow all collectively wrong on the subject.

The majority of adrenal fatigue patients will at times have snap-shot readings that are normal, when blood tested for cortisol levels and they will also pass the ACTH Stimulation Test (confirms or rules out full blown adrenal insufficiency) and is why it is recommended to get multiple readings throughout the day, via saliva cortisol testing for milder forms of adrenal hypo-cortisolism.

When I had the ACTH Stimulation Test performed on me, my cortisol reading was about mid-range on the baseline reading however, I was anxious before and during the test and it's better to get cortisol rhythm of multi-readings during a normal activity day. Even though I had a normal baseline on that ACTH Stimulation Test, I also had a 24 hour urinary test through an Endocrinologist's Office and my cortisol averaged "10.7", with normal range at the lab being <119 for males ages 18 and above. To be in the middle of that one (mid-range), I would have had to have a result of about a 50 or 60 and my Dr. admitted it was a very low reading for a 24 hour urine cortisol test. This confirmed I didn't have true, full-blown adrenal insufficiency but that I did have a serious case of adrenal fatigue.

In research articles, where patients with different diseases, are found to have low cortisol levels, the medical investigators are usually referring to "low cortisol" as being in the low-normal range, so is low compared to "controls" and low compared to normal subjects. They even give the number differences, calling them "significant" even when the difference is only 2 or 3 points lower than normal subjects have.

One statement the NIH makes in their Centers For Disease Control study of CFS, that has always stuck with me is this one; "Doctors have long known that even subtle deficiencies in cortisol is associated with lethargy and fatigue" (Oct, 1996).

I've lately come more to the conclusion that I've suspected from the beginning of researching on adrenal fatigue, that supplementing with DHEA, will help low DHEA levels but usually doesn't help with low cortisol. Maybe in some patients it does help to raise cortisol, once the circle of conversion goes completely around but there's conflicting info about DHEA out there.

What will help the adrenals to produce more cortisol, are vitamins that support adrenal function, rest and adequate sleep and if needed, the safe and cautious use of licorice extract and adrenal glandular extracts.

Some Doctors also sometimes prescribe; pregnenolone to adrenal fatigue patients or other combinations of hormones. A lot of medical resources say that the majority of women can safely take 25mg or less of DHEA and there is very low risk of it causing their androgen levels (male hormones) to go too high and men are supposed to be able to take up to 50mg safely.

I don't feel DHEA would suppress cortisol to a significant degree at these doses but the point is that they also might not help raise cortisol, so that taking it alone, could cause more of a DHEA to cortisol ratio imbalance. This isn't true of people who have low DHEA but normal cortisol levels because DHEA is all they need in these cases. The Journal of Pharmacology has a research article that states that patients with Crohn's Disease and Lupus, are one example of low DHEA.

When the hormone is supplemented in these cases, it improves symptoms of these diseases but DHEA can become low for other reasons as well.

The "American Psychiatric Association", made a statement in the "American Journal of Psychiatry", in a research test that was conducted by 3 psychiatrists and 6 MDs. They stated that supplementing Post Traumatic Stress Disorder patients (PTSD) with low-dose cortical can help them because they found that the low cortisol found in this condition, is a major factor in symptoms. This study, which didn't go overboard with the dosing of cortisol, like others have, such as those experimenting with cortisol supplementing in CFS patients, had more favorable results that are promising for future studies.

There are now studies reported by the major medical research publishing groups that show that CFS patients did improve with lower-dose cortisol treatment. These studies are newer than the ones where they reported "adrenal suppression" and other adverse effects at higher dose treatment.

A Complete Look at CFS and Fibromyalgia

Cortisol replacement therapy is only available by prescription, by a licensed medical professional but hopefully as more research is done, they will find a safe dose that will help treat adrenal fatigue type syndromes.

CHAPTER FIVE

Epstein-Barr Virus and Chronic Fatigue Syndrome

One major virus that other NIH studies have concluded as being highly associated with CFS, which also has low cortisol as a feature, is the Epstein-Barr Virus which causes mononucleosis.

I had a severe case of mononucleosis as a kid, at about age-10 and have always believed there is a connection of it, to both my thyroid disease and CFS.

When I was optimized on HRT but continued to have symptoms, some that were not typical of thyroid, including the following:

• severe post exertion malaise
• swollen neck lymph nodes
• orthostatic hypotension (dizzy when first standing)
• chemical sensitivities

I decided to get tested for EBV. I had read so much about research that suggests the possibility that EBV like others in the herpes virus family, can flare-up in persons with a compromised or deficient immune system (immune dysfunction). My EBV/IGG result was "218" with the normal range being <20 (less than twenty). This means my EBV count was more than 10 times the normal cut-off range.

While a large percent of the population tests positive for EBV (statistics estimate 80%), titers as high as mine are not common, unless a person is actually experiencing active mononucleosis. In my case, I feel the EBV has a connection to both my Hashimoto's Thyroiditis and CFS. The NIH also has research published on the PubMed website that associates EBV with autoimmune thyroiditis.

The Epstein-Barr Virus (EBV) subject is one of real interest to me, especially since searching and researching on the subject. I found lots of medical studies that associate EBV with lots of conditions and diseases not the least of which is Chronic Fatigue Syndrome/CFS.

A few of these studies state that in people with deficiencies in their immune systems, the virus can "reactivate" (re-surge in phases) and also "replicate" (increase in phases).

Not many doctors recognize these facts but they are true non-the-less and EBV has been linked to causing autoimmune diseases as well, such as autoimmune thyroid diseases.

In my opinion, EBV has been active in my system since having my having mononucleosis as a child. I also believe it is responsible for my autoimmune thyroid disease (Hashimoto's thyroiditis). Another interesting fact is sub-clinical to moderate thyroid hormone deficiency being found commonly in people with CFS.

My lymph glands in my neck swell as well and feel mildly sore, in phases and have at least a mild swelling in them all of the time. My CFS symptoms also flare in phases and these can be more severe when I work extra hard or experience increased stress.

Here are quotes/links I find interesting on this subject:

Research quote – Oxford Journals:

"Reactivation of EBV infection is a common finding in immunocompromised individuals."

Research link>
http://ndt.oxfordjournals.org/cgi/content/abstract/12/10/2099

Research Quote – U.S. NIH:

"Although the symptoms of infectious mononucleosis usually resolve in 1 or 2 months, EBV remains dormant or latent in a few cells in the throat and blood for the rest of the person's life. Periodically, the virus can reactivate and is commonly found in the saliva of infected persons. This reactivation usually occurs without symptoms of illness....It is important to note that symptoms related to infectious mononucleosis caused by EBV infection seldom last for more than 4 months. When such an illness lasts more than 6 months, it is frequently called chronic EBV infection.

However, valid laboratory evidence for continued active EBV infection is seldom found in these patients. The illness should be investigated further to determine if it meets the criteria for chronic fatigue syndrome, or CFS. This process includes ruling out other causes of chronic illness or fatigue."

Research link>>
http://www.cdc.gov/ncidod/diseases/ebv.htm
(U.S. National Institutes of Health - Centers for Disease Control – reprints allowed for public education purposes.)

More in regard to the connection of EBV to both CFS and Fibromyalgia will be included in Chapter Seven.

CHAPTER SIX

My Own Diagnosis of Thyroid Disease, CFS and Adrenal Fatigue

One of the reasons I wish to include a chapter on my personal story is because of my thyroid disease aspect. Medical sources, including the National Institutes of Health (U.S.) have published medical research that strongly associates thyroid diseases, especially the autoimmune types, to Fibromyalgia.

There are also many thyroid patients who experience co-morbid CFS or a mix of both CFS and Fibromyalgia. One such person is well known Thyroid Patient Advocate Mary Shomon, who has written a book, as a result of experiencing these syndromes co-morbid to her thyroid disease, entitled "Living Well with Chronic Fatigue Syndrome and Fibromyalgia".

My ongoing battle with adrenal fatigue began to manifest even before I experienced the obvious onset of Hashimoto's/Hypothyroidism in early 2003.

I began to notice months previous to diagnosis
that my tolerance for stress and my recuperative
abilities, to spring back from hard physical
activity, illnesses, excessive stressors etc.., was
slowly diminishing. When my hypothyroid
disease kicked in, the adrenal fatigue hit a peak of
severity and the combination of the two really
threw me for a loop.

When Chronic Disease is Left Untreated

The first Doctors I went to didn't investigate to
find the thyroid disease and I was not being
treated for it, so in the mean time I had to push
myself incredibly hard just to keep going. I also
had an extremely stressful job in property
management at that time.

Finally at one point, the adrenal fatigue turned
into severe "adrenal exhaustion" and I
experienced a strange viral type illness that left
me with severe hives (these resolved) and swollen
neck lymph-nodes that are swollen to this day!
This is also when my chemical sensitivities
became much worse to caffeine chocolate, alcohol
and stimulants of any kind.

In other words I had developed increased Multiple Chemical Sensitivities (MCS).

I finally demanded blood tests and as a result, was treated for diagnosed-hypothyroidism but the adrenal fatigue remained, re-occurring in flares of symptoms. Over time, I learned the difference between the symptoms of adrenal fatigue/exhaustion and thyroid symptoms. With adrenal exhaustion, I experience severe post-exertion malaise and it can take a couple of days sometimes to recuperate from hard physical activity.

My CFS and Abnormal TSH Level

In the year 2006, my blood lab results, to monitor my thyroid hormone therapy, including TSH, T-4 and Free T-3 (thyroid function tests), were not jiving or correlating with each other. My TSH, at just below 0.2 (normal range 0.3 to 5.0), did not match up with the thyroid hormone levels which were also low. Usually a low TSH will mean high readings of the thyroid hormones or "hyperthyroidism".

Patients taking Armour Thyroid (brand of T-4/T-3 thyroid med I take) do commonly have a somewhat low T-4 level but usually not flagged below normal and a below normal TSH usually means over-treatment with thyroid medication but this was not true in my case.

My Doctor, an Endocrinologist, actually raised my 120mg dose, to 150mg, so increased it 30mg, despite my low TSH. He said TSH in some patients, does not always accurately reflect some of the other thyroid lab levels. In my case, this was due to my other endocrine glands, including my "pituitary" (regulates the thyroid), also operating at sub-clinically low levels, due to my also having CFS. Many medical sources state that CFS results in a "blunted HPA Axis" (hypothalamus-pituitary-adrenal axis).

CFS is more common in Thyroid Patients

He also said from all of my test results, including low adrenal hormones, a highly elevated Epstein-Barr Virus count, continually swollen lymph nodes in my throat etc..., that I have co-existing Chronic Fatigue Syndrome (CFS).

A Complete Look at CFS and Fibromyalgia

I had already been told this by a chiropractic doctor, three years earlier. He also added that thyroid patients sometimes have multi-endocrine problems, when everything runs low in addition to the thyroid gland but is especially true if the patient also has CFS.

I asked him if CFS was found more commonly in thyroid disease patients and he said it was but is often not recognized by doctors and is sometimes attributed to thyroid treatment failure. This all amazed me because I had seen this Endocrinologist, 4 times previous and I had never asked him if he recognized CFS as a real syndrome/illness.

He said he certainly does and he recognized it in me, without my having ever brought the subject of CFS up to him. Several years following this diagnosis of Hashimoto's and CFS, I have improved in many ways, especially when my thyroid is treated well, which reduces and helps control all symptoms significantly.

The Effect of Thyroid Flares on CFS Symptoms

I also asked my doctor if thyroid patients commonly have symptom flare-ups and he said any patient with autoimmune thyroid disease will have ups and downs with symptoms, due to antibody and inflammation levels fluctuating, which in turn causes thyroid hormones to also fluctuate slightly. I believe this is also an aspect in the symptom-levels of patients with co-morbid CFS and Fibromyalgia.

My doctor ordered follow up blood tests for me after two months on the increased thyroid med dose, asking for TSH, Free T-4 and Free T-3. My TSH was and is consistently below normal with blood retests but must be in my case due to my having co-morbid CFS. This keeps my thyroid hormone levels at mid-range and above, which most treated thyroid patients need to feel well.

Testing for Adrenal Fatigue

I haven't often shared about my struggles with the co-occurring CFS but have done relatively well with it much of the time.

A Complete Look at CFS and Fibromyalgia

I always remain positive about it as I continue to deal with symptoms. I do feel that thyroid patients with ongoing adrenal fatigue could possibly be experiencing a blunted HPA axis and co-morbid CFS. If they suspect they have ongoing adrenal fatigue or CFS symptoms, they should ask for their adrenal hormone levels to be tested, preferably by multiple saliva samples over a 24 hour period, to better determine their cortisol rhythm.

Treating all Contributing Factors

My doctor did say that treating thyroid disease or any other underlying autoimmune condition is a major factor in helping control the symptoms of CFS and I know this has been true in my case. I also take adrenal support when needed that consists of a combination of vitamins, safe herbals and adrenal glandular supplement, which also helps control my symptoms of CFS and the adrenal fatigue that is a major feature of it.

{It is an incorrect view for medical sources to state that having thyroid disease, eliminates the possibility of having CFS because this is not true in some cases.

A Complete Look at CFS and Fibromyalgia

In fact autoimmune diseases including thyroid ones, may be a trigger for causing co-existing CFS or Fibromyalgia. The U.S. NIH has changed on their stance in this regard and now states that CFS can be co morbid to endocrine illnesses.}

Improvements in my Symptoms

Since receiving treatment for these health disorders I have seen significant improvement in them. I do still experience flares of symptoms, if I venture outside of a diet restricting stimulants or if I do not keep my stress levels under control. It was my own experience that inspired me to research intensely on the subject of thyroid disease and how CFS and Fibromyalgia are often co-morbid to it.

It is my belief that Chronic Fatigue Syndrome (CFS) has a type of adrenal exhaustion involved with it (one major aspect) and that adrenal fatigue can be a forerunner to it in some cases. The most well-established feature of CFS that you find in medical research (also Fibromyalgia), is "low cortisol levels".

I do not believe this is a coincidence but something that makes sense because the main purposes of cortisol is regulating stress and controlling inflammatory responses in the body. Two of the doctors I have been treated by since 2003, also diagnosed me with co-morbid CFS.

Healthy Adrenals Contribute to Healthy Immune Function

The adrenals when low functioning, cause more allergy, viral and illness responses to occur, due to the adrenals role in immune system function, being greatly diminished. Cortisol is also our body's natural anti-inflammatory and so low levels give rise to joint & muscle pain and other inflammatory reactions in the body. All of these factors combined, contribute to the symptoms of adrenal fatigue, CFS and Fibromyalgia and can add to the symptom struggles of hypothyroid patients who have these co-morbid conditions.

CHAPTER SEVEN

More about CFS, Fibromyalgia and Low Cortisol

For more than twenty years, researchers studying Chronic Fatigue Syndrome (CFS) and Fibromyalgia Syndrome, have conducted studies in regard to adrenal function in patients with these syndromes and have concluded that patients are found to be experiencing "low adrenal function" as one of the features of these syndromes. This co-existing condition is also called "adrenal fatigue", "adrenal exhaustion" and "low adrenal reserve".

Through testing of a patient's adrenal hormones, it can be determined if that person has low-functioning adrenals. In addition to blood testing, saliva tests are also accurate for testing the "free levels" of the adrenal hormones, the main ones being DHEA and cortisol. A "24 hour urinary cortisol test" can also be done to test adrenal-cortisol levels.

Another major adrenal function blood test is also available, called the "ACTH Stimulation Test".

This one is designed to confirm or rule out true "adrenal insufficiency" (full blown). Most CFS and Fibromyalgia patients do not have true, full blown adrenal insufficiency but a milder form of adrenal fatigue/exhaustion.

Medical Research - The Effect of CFS and FMS on Cortisol Levels

Research conclusions by major Medical Research groups, including the NIH, state that low cortical levels, are found to be a contributing factor in CFS/FMS, due to dysfunction of the HPA Axis (Hypothalamus-Pituitary-Adrenal Axis).

It is my opinion because of this, that CFS/FMS has as one of its features, a form of adrenal fatigue, that does not meet the definition for true "adrenal insufficiency" and because of this, it cannot be medically treated the same.

With full blown Adrenal Insufficiency, a much more serious condition, the low adrenal hormones must be replaced through steroid treatment (cortisone-steroid/hydrocortisone).

With lesser forms of low adrenal function, such as adrenal fatigue, steroid treatment can possibly worsen the adrenal problem because the steroids may cause "adrenal suppression", which means the patient may have to take the steroids, the rest of their life because anything less than very short-term use of the steroids, can cause this suppression.

Triggers for CFS and FMS

Some of the other things Medical Researchers have studied in regard to CFS and Fibromyalgia, is the fact that these syndromes can have different triggers for different patients but for many, it is an underlying viral, autoimmune, bacterial etc..., type infection in the body, that causes chronic activation of the immune system and over time, this uses up some of the adrenal reserves because the adrenals have a major role in releasing cortisol, the body's natural anti-inflammatory, attempting to ward off inflammation.

Cortisol (also called "cortical"), is also the "stress hormone", that helps the body to deal with stresses of all kinds.

A Complete Look at CFS and Fibromyalgia

Without it, even the smallest stressor would cause shock and death (adrenal crises). It, along with adrenaline, are "fight or flight" hormones and help protect the body from the effects of stress, from minor emotional stress, to major ones, such as a car accident or serious disease.

Diminished Tolerance to Stressors

This in my opinion is why persons with CFS/FMS have such low tolerance for stressors both emotional and physical. With low adrenal function, even mild emotional and physical stresses result in major fatigue, couple this with the immune system dysfunction that CFS/FMS patients also have and you have syndromes with serious symptoms! It may be that the immune deficiency found in both CFS and Fibromyalgia is also a type of burn-out of that system, due to constant, ongoing activation of it, that the body eventually loses the ability to continue.

As with all other opinions about CFS and Fibromyalgia, we have to consider all of the preceeding views, as some of the many theories that are out there.

A Complete Look at CFS and Fibromyalgia

I feel however, that the evidence of low adrenal function in CFS and Fibromyalgia is overwhelming. What I have described, is what I feel connects these syndromes to a form of adrenal fatigue.

Stress is a known trigger for adrenal fatigue and related syndromes, such as Chronic Fatigue Syndrome and Fibromyalgia and it can also bring an autoimmune disease to the surface, that is in the body but hasn't fully manifested and thyroid diseases are some of the more common ones that are triggered by stress, especially Grave's Disease/hyperthyroidism.

PTSD (Post Traumatic stress Disorder) is also a chronic stress caused syndrome as mentioned previously but is also classified as an anxiety disorder.

Chronic Stressors – A Precursor to Stress Related Syndromes

I personally went through an extreme, chronic time of stress and my thyroid disease, called "Hashimoto's Thyroiditis" and adrenal fatigue manifested because of it.

A Complete Look at CFS and Fibromyalgia

I was untreated for several months and the result was an added severe flare-up I experienced, that I know for a fact triggered an even more severe CFS form of adrenal fatigue in me (Chronic Fatigue syndrome).

I initially developed severe hives and a strange viral type illness that left me with the CFS. After this, the lymph nodes in my neck remained swollen to this day and I have severe chemical sensitivities.

My belief is that CFS is an altered HPA Axis ("blunted"), plus altered immune function syndrome combined, so I do try to tell people to get their adrenal hormones and all other hormones checked as well, including the sex hormones because it is my belief that hormonal imbalances over time, can possibly result in CFS and Fibromyalgia type illnesses.

Some who read my articles or have read my posts on forums, may wonder why I have the passion I do for the adrenal subjects.

It is because it is my belief that adrenal fatigue can contribute to the development of CFS and/or FMS type syndromes, when not taken seriously and investigated/treated if a patient has it.

Working Toward Recovery

Things that speed recovery for CFS include:

• treating the adrenal fatigue
• getting a lot of sleep and rest
• a healthy diet
• exercising to tolerance
• making sure other diseases a patient might have are treated properly

Under-treatment of a thyroid disorder for example, can serve as a trigger for CFS flare-ups and may actually be a trigger for the syndrome itself according to some medical sources.

For many with CFS, chronic stress was a trigger for the onset of the syndrome.

CHAPTER EIGHT

The Connection of Epstein-Barr Virus to CFS and Fibromyalgia

The EBV (Epstein-Barr Virus), which causes Mononucleosis initially in some patients can afterward, remain in a persons body for life. This virus is suspected of having a strong connection to CFS. While most people with EBV in their system (estimates are 80 to 95% of the population), only have antibody titers to the virus, that are just barely positive, like a "5", a "10", "20" above normal, etc..., others actually have flare-ups of this virus, probably due to a compromised immune system (immune deficiency) that causes really high counts/titers of the virus to increase in their bodies over time.

Many in the medical field are of the opinion that EBV is a background virus like many others in the herpes virus-family, that can flare-up like cold sores can (also a herpes virus). When flare-ups happen, they believe it causes or at least contributes to symptoms of CFS.

In my case, my EBV count was "218" with normal range being <20, so mine was more than ten times the normal cut off range.

EBV – An Indicator of Immune Function

Some Doctors believe the EBV test means nothing, unless actually being used to test for Mononucleosis but there has to be a reason some patient's EBV counts elevate so highly. Both MDs I now go to, believe that EBV can flare-up in some patients who have high titers of it. Many sources also state that adrenal fatigue is a major feature of this because the adrenals are the major moderators of our immune system.

While EBV may not be the actual root cause of CFS, it has been shown to be an indicator of immune dysfunction in studies that have been conducted. In my opinion, it is just one of many factors that can contribute to the symptoms of CFS. In addition to EBV, other herpes-family viruses suspected in the cause of CFS and Fibromyalgia include the human herpes virus 6 (HHV-6), Cytomegalovirus (also a herpes virus) and Coxsackie viruses B1 and B4.

CHAPTER NINE

More on Symptoms and Diagnosis of Fibromyalgia

Widespread and Chronic Muscle Pain

Fibromyalgia is a syndrome of widespread body pain and fatigue. There are signs and symptoms that can help to identify and diagnose Fibromyalgia.

People with Fibromyalgia syndrome (FMS) will find that they experience widespread and severe body pain that is chronic (ongoing). The pain will affect the muscles and joints but will also produce "tender points." These are places on the body that experience pain when pressure is applied to them, where muscles are attached to bones, at the joints. Some in the medical community vary in their opinions as to whether FMS is a rheumatic condition or strictly a pain syndrome. Others believe it is a combination of both.

Published Diagnostic Criteria

In addition to also being recognized as an inflammatory disorder, some research studies have also found that FMS may be an autoimmune-related disorder. Some medical research groups have also found that FMS and Chronic Fatigue Syndrome (CFS) have 75% crossover symptom similarities as mentioned previously.

Some published diagnostic studies have suggested that Fibromyalgia is better determined when a person experiencing FMS symptoms is found to have at least 11 of the 18 possible tender points that can occur throughout the body. These are areas where pain will occur upon applying mild pressure to them, using a fingertip.

The areas on the body where these tender points may occur include the following:

• the hips

• the knees
...

...

• the back of the head near the base of the neck

• upper areas of the chest

• the upper back in the cervical spine area

• the elbows

• the shoulders

Fatigue and Sleep Disturbances

Fatigue is another major symptom of FMS and it is sometimes exacerbated by sleep disturbances that can also occur. The fatigue is often relentless and proper sleep and rest does little to alleviate it completely.

Normal circadian sleep rhythms (cycles) that are supposed to occur become abnormal in Fibromyalgia patients, which results in daytime sleepiness and feeling more awake during nighttime hours.

Medical research, including that conducted by the National Institutes of Health (U.S.-NIH), suggests that abnormal functioning of the adrenal glands is one possible cause of the disrupted sleep patterns, due to the adrenal hormone "cortisol" not being properly regulated by the adrenal glands in people who have Fibromyalgia.

Digestive Disturbances and IBS

FMS patients may complain of severe indigestion, heartburn and acid reflux with FMS but may also experience alternating spells of constipation and diarrhea. This may indicate that they are also suffering from Irritable Bowel Syndrome (IBS). Frequent gastritis and bloating may also manifest as part of the digestive problems that can occur with Fibromyalgia.

Headaches and Sensory Disturbances

Many people with Fibromyalgia experience frequent headaches and these may have a neurological aspect to them that they have not experienced previously.

The headaches may sometimes have an unusual pattern to them or will affect the person's senses as they occur (i.e. eyesight, sense of smell, taste and hearing). These sensory changes can occur with headaches or may also occur without them.

These may include heightened and/or loss of sensitivity to the following:

• light

• noises

• flavors

• odors

• sense of touch

Emotional and Mental Symptoms

People with FMS may also experience symptoms of anxiety and depression and a change in mental functioning. These emotional symptoms may alternate between those of anxiety and depression.

The patient may experience mostly one of these mood problems, rather than a mix of them. A person with Fibromyalgia may experience anxiety symptoms as an increase in chronic worry and episodes of fear, including the possibility of panic attacks. The depression may be perceived by them as a profound sadness, an emptiness or hopelessness.

This demonstrates the importance in monitoring Fibromyalgia patients for any signs of worsening emotional symptoms, which may require treatment as a separate issue, in addition to treatments that are needed for rheumatic symptoms (muscle pain).

Mental functioning may also become diminished in Fibromyalgia patients. They may have difficulty concentrating and will experience what is often referred to as "brain fog," a term to describe mental dullness or an inability to focus with the same sharpness they had previous to their illness. Short-term memory loss is also experience in some FMS patients.

See Your Doctor

People who experience the symptoms described in the subheadings above need to see a qualified, licensed medial physician in order to confirm a diagnosis of Fibromyalgia or other conditions with similar symptoms. Patients receiving a diagnosis of FMS can move forward with appropriate treatment, which can help to control symptoms or diminish them significantly and return them to an improved quality of life.

CHAPTER TEN

More on the Suspected Causes of CFS

Triggers for Chronic Fatigue Syndrome

Decades of medical research on Chronic Fatigue Syndrome has revealed a number of abnormalities in patients with the syndrome. One definitive cause has yet to be found.

Chronic Fatigue Syndrome (CFS) is a complicated and sometimes mysterious illness. Medical research studies have been ongoing for many years in attempts to find a definitive cause for the illness. Medical groups studying CFS have instead found a number of aspects of the syndrome that are clearly present but each may play a role or be one of the many factors of CFS rather than its definitive cause.

Post Viral Illness

A number of viruses studied in relation to CFS have been found to be present in significant titers (lab result measurements) in people suffering the syndrome.

Among the viruses suspected of being possible causes or triggers for CFS, are enteroviruses and retroviruses. These include the Epstein-Barr Virus (EBV) that is usually contracted during childhood and carried throughout one's lifetime, human herpesvirus 6 and the Cytomegalovirus. Candida albican overgrowth (fungal/yeast infection), although not in the virus category has also been suspected as a possible cause or trigger for CFS.

Some of these viruses, including EBV cause no symptoms in most people when contracted (can potentially cause mononucleosis) but will increase in the number of titers found in the blood when the virus replicates.

It has been proposed as a possibility that the increased replication of viruses may occur when the immune system is not functioning well in suppressing their ability to replicate or reactivate. Reactivation would mean that a virus resurges at times, causing repeated illness in the infected person who has not fully developed immunity to it.

Imbalance in the Involuntary Nervous System

In other studies of CFS patients, they have been found to be experiencing dysfunction in their involuntary nervous systems (INS), also referred to as "autonomic failure" and "dysautonomia".

The INS is responsible for regulating blood pressure with changes in physical activity and changes in positions of the body (i.e. sitting, standing and lying flat). It also regulates all other involuntary bodily functions, including respiration, digestion, kidney function, liver function, etc… and increases these functions when needed (sympathetic response) or decreases them (parasympathetic response).

An imbalance in this system will cause these functions to be inadequate at times and over-responsive at other times. If for example, physical activity is increased and blood pressure needs to rise but fails to do so, this can result in bodily fatigue due to a lack of needed blood flow to the muscles and organs of the body.

If bodily functions need to decrease at times of rest or when sleep is needed but remain highly activated this will result in fatigue as well.

Dysfunction of the Immune System

Other, conclusions resulting from medical studies of CFS causes, has found that patients with the syndrome are experiencing a dysfunction of the immune system. The immunity or what might be referred to as "resistance" to viruses and allergens is greatly diminished in CFS patients.

This means that the body is more susceptible to viruses and allergens and recovers more slowly from exposure and infections to them, than are people with healthy immune systems.

Infections of these types can cause a mild systemic (system-wide) inflammation in the body and cause the person experiencing them, to feel as if they are experiencing perpetual flu-like symptoms or a continual low-grade fever.

Chronic Stress

CFS patients often report in medical study questionnaires that they experienced severe, prolonged or traumatic stress, just before the onset of their CFS symptoms. Stress is responded-to by the part of the endocrine system called the "HPA Axis", standing for the Hypothalamus-Pituitary-Adrenal gland system. When chronic stress is experienced, this system is hyper-active and over time, becomes "blunted", meaning it becomes fatigued or diminished in its ability to run at overdrive. This causes slower release of the hormones that come from these endocrine glands that work in sync (full-circle) to supply the body with stress coping abilities.The end result of the hypothalamus stimulating the pituitary gland, which then in-turn stimulates the adrenal glands, is the release of the stress hormone "cortisol". When this system becomes blunted after extended hyperactivity, cortisol levels begin to fall or what is sometimes referred to as "hypocortisolemia" or "hypoadrenia". Some sources recognizing this mild form of adrenal dysfunction refer to it as "Adrenal Fatigue".

CHAPTER ELEVEN

Treatments for CFS and Fibromyalgia

There have been no cures found for either of these syndromes and so the treatments are to reduce the symptoms of them. Some patients do see complete recovery but there is no solid medically confirmed proof that treatment of the symptoms is what brought recovery in these cases.

Since the symptoms of these two syndromes crossover significantly, let me first mention the specific treatment for Fibromyalgia patients who have significantly severe muscle and joint pain. Following that, I will list the treatments that are commonly administered for both syndromes.

Fibromyalgia patients are often given medications to control the pain in their muscles and joints. Some are also given anti-inflammatory drugs, to reduce inflammation that can also occur and that can contribute to the pain symptoms. These include over-the-counter and prescription pain and anti-inflammatory medications and corticosteroids (hydrocortisone), also called glucocorticoids.

A Complete Look at CFS and Fibromyalgia

Treatments that are commonly administered for both syndromes include correction of hormonal, vitamin, mineral and nutritional deficiencies of any kind, found through thorough blood lab testing. Hormones that may be low in these syndromes include:

• thyroid
• adrenal
• sex

Correction of these can significantly improve symptoms, as can correction of any other important body elements (i.e. minerals and nutrients) that may be found to be low.

Some patients see improvement in both emotional and physical symptoms when administered SSRI antidepressants. A therapy called "Cognitive Behavioral Therapy" (CBT) can also be successful in relieving symptoms in some patients, as well as giving them skills for coping with their illness.

Since Adrenal Fatigue (low cortisol) is a major feature of these syndromes, the following treatment recommended for this stress-related aspect, can also improve symptoms significantly.

Get more Sleep, Rest and Relaxation

In today's fast-paced society, a busy schedule can leave little time for adequate sleep, rest and relaxation. This lack of rest can heighten your stress level and place too much demand on the adrenal glands. Like any organ or gland of the body, the adrenals need time to rest in order to rebuild their reserves and abilities to function at optimal level. The job of these glands is to supply the body with adequate levels of adrenal hormones, but they can only do this if the body in general is allowed to rest and relax for sufficient periods of time.

Medical sources state that most people need a minimum of eight hours of sleep per night in order to function at their best level during the daytime and in order for the cells of the body to have adequate time to repair and restore from normal use of the body.

63

Our everyday routines also place a degree of
stress upon our minds and emotions. While sleep
is very important to get in adequate amounts, so is
simple rest and relaxation in general.

If you don't allow for leisure time and time to
simply sit or lie down and rest on occasion, you
will not be allowing your body and mind to
unwind from the stressors of everyday duties and
this leads to that feeling of being "stressed out"
by the end of the day or even before the end of the
day.

People with full time jobs are many times actually
required by their employers to provide them two
breaks per day, to take a short rest of usually 20
minutes per break. This is due to studies that
indicate even short rest periods help workers
rejuvenate their energies, in order to continue and
complete their work days more efficiently.

Rest, sleep and relaxation are also necessary to
prevent or recover from adrenal fatigue.

A Complete Look at CFS and Fibromyalgia

Reduce your Stress Levels

No one living in the world today can escape or be immune to stress. Stress is a fact of life; our goal is to work on reducing its effects and learn coping skills, so that we find ways to eliminate as much of it as we possibly can. The adrenal glands help us to cope with and to recover from stress by providing the body with adequate levels of the stress hormone "cortisol".

This hormone is also considered to be a "fight or flight" hormone, just like adrenaline. But while adrenaline is the more short term energizing hormone needed at times of danger (to escape or fight a situation or enemy), cortisol is the long term fight or flight hormone, giving us the needed flow of energy, throughout the day, to perform our normal tasks.

Relentless and ongoing stress can eventually use up the reserves of this hormone faster than the adrenals are able to supply it, unless we allow ourselves time to recuperate from stress.

Only then can the adrenals rebuild the reserves of this very important stress hormone and the others it also supplies to the body. Stress can be reduced simply by resting and giving ourselves time during each day to unwind for a few minutes at a time.

It is also important not to get uptight throughout the day over small problems that arise. We should learn to not take the smaller problems as seriously, because there are potentially too many of them that can arise and this will keep our stress levels peaked too often or for extended periods.

In addition to taking "timeouts" to unwind during the day, we can also involve ourselves in hobbies or leisure activities that give us pleasure during our times away from work, further helping us to relax and unwind. Involving yourself in enjoyable activities can provide you with much needed enjoyment-of-life that helps you relieve stress and feel more refreshed when the time for work returns.

Take Supplements that help Strengthen the Adrenals

There are many supplements that can be taken to help keep the body and adrenal glands healthy and strengthened so they can handle the everyday stress life brings upon all of us. A really good multi-vitamin is always a great idea and there are many good ones out there to choose from. Some major vitamin companies actually make vitamins called "stress formulas" or "stress tabs" and these contain the vitamins and minerals that help the body cope with and recover from stress.

Additional vitamin supplements in particular that are very helpful to the adrenal glands include "B" vitamins – in particular, B-12, B-5 and B-6. Vitamin "C" is also an important vitamin for healthy adrenal function. Minerals that can help with adrenal function include zinc and magnesium. There are also adrenal herbal formulas that contain helpful supplements, but these should be researched carefully by anyone who is considering taking them.

They should also discussed with your doctor before taking them. Purchase supplements only from reliable, reputable companies.

Other natural supplements to be taken after observing these precautions include "adrenal glandular" (usually beef source), "licorice root extract" (helps adrenals produce more cortisol) and DHEA (over-the-counter adrenal hormone). Some Adrenal Fatigue sufferers also report improvement using herbal and other energy supplements such as Ashwagandha, Ginseng, Ribrose and Co-Q10.

All of these supplements can potentially be helpful, but everyone is unique; some supplements work better for some than others and sometimes it simply takes a trial of several of these to find the one that eventually helps the most. Also make sure you thoroughly research any supplements you plan to take, discuss them with your doctor and only take the manufacture's recommended dose or that set by your doctor.

Incorporate Regular Exercise into your Health Regimen

Exercise is important in strengthening the body in general. Regular exercise also results in strengthened adrenal glands. Doctors know that exercise helps the hormones in our bodies to do their jobs better because it helps to circulate and metabolize them better. Cortisol, the stress hormone produced by the adrenals, also helps to regulate our glucose (blood sugar) and is one reason exercise helps in this process.

When you begin an exercise routine, it is important that you do so at the pace your body can tolerate. You do not want to overdo on exercise; too much exercise will not increase the benefit from it faster, but can actually have an adverse effect. This is especially true of people who are already experiencing adrenal fatigue. They can have reduced tolerance for exercise and if they do not pace themselves, they can worsen the adrenal fatigue rather than helping resolve it.

Walking is one of the best exercises to start out with, and a good everyday exercise for anyone.

Some who start with walking can eventually progress to jogging, if that's what they chose and they are healthy enough to do so. If you prefer walking as your exercise, many sources state that walking 15 to 20 minutes at least three times a week will provide a healthy benefit, and five times or more per week increases that benefit.

See a licensed professional - medical practitioner when seeking the diagnosis and treatment of Chronic Fatigue Syndrome or Fibromyalgia.

(END)